Rebirth of an Academic Hospital Department

Experiences from the First Year

JACOB ROSENBERG, MD.

Copyright © 2013 Jacob Rosenberg

All rights reserved.

ISBN:1491298316
ISBN-13: 978-1491298312

CONTACT INFO

Jacob Rosenberg, MD, DSc, FACS
Professor, Head of department
Herlev Hospital – University of Copenhagen
Department of Surgery
Herlev Ringvej 75 - DK-2730 Herlev –
Denmark
e-mail: jacob.rosenberg@regionh.dk

CONTENTS

	Preface	iii
1	Why did I write this book?	1
2	Situation at take-over	4
3	Kick off	8
4	Clear mission statement	9
5	Who is the boss?	10
6	A new atmosphere	12
7	Changes in the surgical wards	13
8	Patient satisfaction	15
9	Ambulatory polyclinic	17
10	Endoscopy unit	20
11	Organization of acute functions	22
12	Reorganizing the booking of surgical procedures	24

13	Room changes	26
14	Economy – problems and solutions	27
15	What can they expect from me?	30
16	Time plan for the new department	32
17	Production and innovation	33
18	It is ok to be the best	36
19	New professors	37
20	Financial recovery	38
21	What is next?	42
22	Summary of changes	43
23	Conclusion	46
24	Thank you	48
25	Further reading	49

PREFACE

I want to be honest with you: This is my first e-book and I have to get used to this new format. I have written hundreds of scientific papers through the years and my first idea with the present manuscript was to write it as a formal article to be published in an indexed journal. However, after thinking it through for a while, it was obvious that the content of the book would be more personal and experience-based rather than "scientific" with the need of a comprehensive literature base with lots of references. Thus, the result was this e-book where there is more room for sharing personal experiences and good advices to the reader. I sincerely hope that you find the content usable.

April 2013, Jacob Rosenberg.

1 WHY DID I WRITE THIS BOOK?

The correct question may in fact be how am i qualified to tell anyone how to run an academic department at a university hospital?
I have only been head of department for a year and I have no formal education in management or leadership. I am a general surgeon and have for about 10 years been a full professor of surgery at the university of copenhagen. This job consists of half time clinical work and half time research and teaching. As a consultant surgeon there are of course some leadership tasks during the daily routines, but of course not at the level of a department head. In the research part of my position as a professor I have for years run my own research group and in that context gained experience with mentoring and inspiring younger colleagues for better performances.
When the position was available as head of department i had some ideas of how to run a big academic department and apparently the hospital directors were impressed enough to hire me for this position.

I should also say that in my country it is not normal that clinical departments are run by academic professors since running a department is normally looked on as a task that requires almost 100% administrative work with no room for academic "playing around" with research and teaching. I thought this through thoroughly before applying for the position and decided that I should show them otherwise. With firm and insisting delegation of responsibilities and tasks to people in the department I was sure that it could work and hopefully with better satisfaction for the employees.

In fact I think that it has been a big advantage to be an academic person, at least in the beginning of the administration period in the department, because the employees would not question my clinical skills. At the same time it is natural for a new leader to get a certain period of calmness to show some results on the economical and management side of the running of the department. This made a very good starting position for me and i have been lucky enough to actually show some good results during this first year.

As mentioned above I did not have any experience of running such a big unit when I started in this job and therefore I now after a year chose to write up my experiences in an e-book, so that others in a similar position may hopefully pick up some good advices from this. I did not have anyone to guide me in detail in the beginning, and I would actually have liked to have a book like this at hand when I started.

2 SITUATION AT TAKE-OVER

The gastroenterology unit has a total of 90 beds of which 14 belongs to the medical gastroenterological section of the department. The other 76 beds belong to the surgical section. Surgery comprises only abdominal surgery, whereas breast, thyroid, orthopedic etc. Have their own departments. The accrual area is for basic diagnoses such as gallbladders and hernias around 480.000 citizens corresponding to approximately 10% of the population of Denmark. For certain special diagnoses the accrual area consists of 2.5 million people corresponding to 50% of the country. A busy night would easily consist of 30 acute admissions of which maybe 5-10 would need acute surgery during the evening and night hours. Thus, in the evening and night hours we have 2 interns, 2 residents and 1 consultant in the hospital and 1 more on call from home. Because of very strict rules from the medical association around duty hours we have to have quite a few physicians and surgeons employed in the department. Thus, we have at the moment 75 surgeons and physicians employed, including interns and residents. The total staff in the department comprises a little less than 400 heads including both full time and part time employees. We run a ward specialized for acute admissions, two stationary surgical wards and one with medical patients, day surgery at two different hospitals and surgery for inpatients at one hospital. Besides this we have an advanced endoscopy unit with 6 endoscopy rooms. They do gastroscopies, sigmoideoscopies, colonoscopies, ERCPs, endoscopic ultrasound and various other advanced endoscopic procedures. Both surgeons and gastroenterologists perform advanced endoscopic procedures in our unit.

Previous leadership

Leadership of a clinical department in our country consists of a head surgeon or physician and a head nurse. The previous head surgeon was a kind person and also a skilled surgeon, but he was maybe not so keen to delegate the responsibility to other people. All decisions therefore had to go through him and, although i am sure that it was not intentional, it probably produced much focus on details and less on the bigger development lines for the department. Furthermore, he did not include the head nurse in the economical decisions.

The economical situation was a bit out of control. For instance every month about 90.000 US $ were paid for extra time for the surgeons (in total). This amount was not in the budget so it was certainly a challenge when I took over to get the spending under control.

There was general tiredness among the medical/surgical and nursing staff during the last couple of years. It is not fair to blame the former chief for this, but it may be a simple phenomenon caused by having the same management in a department like this for more than 10 years. In previous years the department had been famous for big open surgical procedures such as liver- and pancreatic surgery, but a re-structuring of surgical care in the whole country resulted in movement of these procedures to another hospital. I have been one of the pioneers of minimal invasive surgery in our country, and therefore was at the right place at the right time to help with the growth of minimal invasive surgery in our department.

Conclusion

I may have had some good ideas and also with close collaboration with the head nurse and the staff in general been able to make a positive turn-around in the department. I have in fact also to some extend been at the right place at the right time. The department needed a change of management after many years of focus on big open surgical procedures. Thus, it was time for a change, and I was lucky enough to be given this challenge.

3 KICK OFF

Before starting in the new job as head of the department we had a one day seminar at another location. The people included in this were the head nurse, myself and a senior surgeon from the department who had also previously been a department head for many years in another hospital. This was a very productive day where we discussed all areas of the department and all the plans for changes. The plans were adjusted so that when this day was over the three of us were absolutely 100% in agreement of everything. Part of the management strategy (see below) was to have a clear and rock steady mission for the department, so there would not be any room for disagreement in the top management team.

Then about a week after take over the head nurse and myself held a presentation in one of the large lecture halls in the hospital for the entire staff, where we presented how we looked at things and our plans for changes. It was our impression that the staff had looked forward to this event and the atmosphere was quite positive.

4 CLEAR MISSION STATEMENT

As mentioned above the plan was to give a very clear mission statement from the head nurse and myself to the entire staff. In this way we communicated that we would enhance patient satisfaction, have better and more research, better education and a firm focus on quality of care in all areas of the department. In this way we wanted to create the best department in the country. It was communicated without any doubt that we would not go for the second best. At the same time, however, we of course have to say that we could not achieve this right from the beginning, especially because of the very big economical problems that we were facing, but the goal would still be the same and that was to strive for the very best.

5 WHO IS THE BOSS? MAKING A CLEAR MANAGEMENT HIERARCHY

When I started in the position of head of the department it was my clear impression that much of the dissatisfaction among the staff was due to lack of influence and lack of control of the working conditions. It has therefore been a clear strategy from the start to delegate as much responsibility as possible to the next management level in the hierarchy. At take over we in fact did not have clearly defined middle managers in all parts of the department and therefore the first thing to do was to appoint middle managers in all areas.

The first thing to do was to appoint a daily chief of surgery and a daily chief of medicine. These two persons are clinically skilled and serve a lot of respect from their colleagues. The choice was therefore natural and they control all the daily problems with starting and running the production. In all the clinical areas of the department we have appointed management teams consisting of a doctor and a nurse. They have the full responsibility for ensuring both income and keeping expenses within their limits. They have the immediate "staff responsibilities" and are also responsible for creating the budgeted income for the department by treating enough patients etc.

The overall purpose of delegating responsibility to the management teams in all the clinical areas of the department has been first of all to give a better job satisfaction and at the same time to be able as top management to control what is actually going on a big department like ours. It is merely impossible for the head nurse and me to be in contact personally with all employees and we therefore have to rely on the middle managers for running the department.

6 A NEW ATMOSPHERE

It has been a define strategy to change the atmosphere in the doctors meetings in the morning and later during the day. I had communicated this clearly to the surgeons at the senior level so that they would participate in discussions of patient cases in a learning atmosphere instead of only pointing at the thing that the juniors had done wrong. It is actually a simple thing to change the discussions to a learning environment instead of a negative atmosphere with only blaming errors on the interns and residents. This may sound obvious but it was not the case before.

.

7 CHANGES IN THE SURGICAL WARDS

In one of the surgical wards the atmosphere was especially bad. Many of the patient complaints came from this specific department. The many reasons were probably problems with nursing management in this ward and the lack of stable surgical expertise in the rounds. These problems were not present in the other wards that thus did not have the same amount of patient complaints. The solution was that we changed the nursing management in the specific ward and appointed a surgical consultant to take care of the ward on a daily basis.

We also changed the name of the ward. The previous name was "Upper abdominal surgery" and we simply changed the name to "Department West". This may seem to be a small thing, but together with a new ward management it signaled to the staff, that we had entered a new period and we therefore expected new behavior from especially the nursing staff towards the patients. The new strong nursing management in this ward has changed the daily routines for the nursing staff in order to raise awareness and competence towards the patients.

In general we have problems with many different computer platforms for different administrative systems, e.g. patient files, blood tests, pathology, microbiology, x-ray etc. This requires that the staff spend quite a long time in front of the computer screen instead of close to the patients. We therefore decided to put the computers in front of every patient room so that the nursing staff did not have to go to the central office to document that their work and could do it right outside the patient room instead. In this way the nursing staff would be more close to the patients instead of spending time in the central office in front of the computer screen. One of the complaints of many of the patients was that they did not see the nursing staff (or the doctors) during daytime, and this new positioning of computers outside every patient room hopefully will help against this problem.

Another problem was that patients arriving for elective surgery, typically the day before operation, would wait quite a long time for nurses and doctors to "install them" in the department. This has been solved by appointing two dedicated receiving-nurses who have the only task of taking care of new patients.

8 PATIENT SATISFACTION

In the last few years our department has had the questionable pleasure of having the absolutely lowest score for patient satisfaction in the whole country. This was a catastrophe and we of course had to take this very seriously.

The first thing to do was from the top management to communicate very friendly that we would not accept this in the future, and that patient satisfaction was the top priority in every aspects of activity in the department. The patients were not dissatisfied actually with quality of medical or surgical care, but the main problems were waiting time and a bad tone especially from the nursing staff to the patients. A few months after take-over of the department we had a full Theme Day with all staff, where we discussed these issues in detail. We also invited a patient who had recently had surgery in our department and he explained very emotionally and in detail what the problems were. Having a patient for this session was a very strong experience and it made a deep impression on all the staff. After this we performed qualitative interviews with both patients and relatives in order to detail even more what the problems could be, and what solutions we could choose in order to change this for the future.

Every month, when we have new staff both in the medical/surgical part as well as nursing staff, the head nurse and I talk to them in detail and underline the necessity to look at our jobs as a service for the patients. We are there to help them and we have to do this with compassion and hopefully also with a smile on our lips. Department problems, problems with the colleagues etc. are not to be solved in the patient rooms but to be discussed elsewhere. They have to remember that even though they had a bad night, too many acute admissions or their colleague is an idiot, then they have to remember, that the person at the other end of the stethoscope may have pancreas cancer and be in a lot more trouble than themselves.

.

9 AMBULATORY POLYCLINIC

We had three major problems here: 1) No timeslots for subacute patients. 2) Not enough capacity to take in patients with hernias and gallstone disease for the first contact. 3) Accrual of patients for research projects.

No timeslots for subacute patients
It is needed to have subacute timeslots for patients from outside, and especially for patients who have been discharged from the surgical ward but still need some contact to the department. In order to have a fast flow through the surgical wards we need to be able to discharge patients and give them maybe an appointment in the day clinic after a few days e.g. for control of wound etc. In order to keep a high patient throughput in the wards it is therefore important to have these subacute timeslots in the day clinic.

Not enough capacity to take in patients with hernias and gallstone disease for the first contact
As discussed later in this book we did not produce enough income especially for hernias

and gall bladders and the main problem was actually the waiting time for first visit. One year ago the time to first visit was more than three months and thereby patients naturally went to other hospitals for treatment. In order to secure a stable income for the department it was therefore very important to get more capacity for first visits for patients with hernias and gallstone disease.

You may look at this as a kind of investment, i.e. we had to spend some money for nurses and doctors taking care of these patients at their first visit in order to ensure a stable income for the department. This meant that we opened another line in the day clinic 4 days a week especially for these patients. Another way to create some capacity would be to change some of the cancer control appointments from meeting a surgeon to be taken care of by a nurse specialist instead. This would free some surgeon time and we will use this as part of the capacity for seeing patients with hernias and gallbladders.

Accrual of patients for research projects

The most important place in the department for accrual of patients for research projects is in the day clinic. Most of the research projects are performed in elective surgical patients and it is the best place to include them in the projects if they can be seen by a research nurse in the day clinic. Our surgical research unit (see later) has two full time research nurses and in order to get a better foothold in the day clinic we intend to change the organization so that three full time research nurses will all together share two positions as a research nurse and one as a day clinic nurse. In this way they will shift being allocated to research assignments or to normal patient care in the day clinic and by this it will be easier to include patients from the day clinic.

10 ENDOSCOPY UNIT

A few months ago we have merged three different endoscopy units to one new big unit in newly built facilities in the hospital. The three previous units consisted of a unit only for surgeons and a unit only for gastroenterologists at our hospital and also another unit at another hospital mainly doing advanced endoscopic procedures. We have been very lucky that the hospital has built this new high-end endoscopy unit for our department and that it has been possible to merge these three independent units into one big unit instead.

However, it naturally created some problems because staff from three different units suddenly had to work together and surgeons had to perform endoscopy in medical patients and gastroenterologists had to do endoscopy in surgical patients. The merging of the nursing staff has been quite uneventful and the reason for this is most likely that the local heads of the endoscopy unit (a chief physician and a department nurse) has spent a lot of time creating a good working atmosphere and teaching the staff the different endoscopic procedures and issues about diseases both in surgery and gastroenterology. We still have a task to fulfill about teaching the gastroenterologists about surgical diseases and teaching the surgeons about gastroenterological diseases in order to make the merging 100% complete.

On the doctors side we have reorganized the staff so that we have four full time specialists only doing endoscopies and the professor of endoscopy is in his clinical work only doing endoscopy as well. By doing this we hope to increase the quality remarkably and also be able to give good teaching opportunities because the ones who are teaching the procedures will be very skilled when they don't do anything else than endoscopy every day. The four full time endoscopists are two surgeons and two gastroenterologists.

11 ORGANIZATION OF ACUTE FUNCTIONS

About 80% of our admissions are acute, but this very big area in the department did not previously have a dedicated leadership. We therefore now have employed a surgical consultant as a team leader, and he is leading the acute team together with a department nurse. We are in the process of reorganizing the work in the acute ward with dedicated consultants and new work planning for the residents and interns in this area as well. The process of developing patient flow planning for about 20 different acute diagnoses has started.

We have dedicated ultrasound specialists who every morning between 8 and 9 will perform abdominal ultrasound examinations on all patients where the diagnosis is unclear. This is not the same as a surgical resident doing his or her own ultrasound examination during the call hours since these fast scannings only can discriminate between few different diagnoses. Instead, the morning scanning round by ultrasound specialists is on a high expertise level and they can also do invasive procedures if needed here.

12 REORGANIZING THE BOOKING OF SURGICAL PROCEDURES

About a year ago we had a prospected deficit in our income of almost 10 million US$ and this was partly due to not doing enough operations.

The effectiveness of the operating department has been and is still to a certain extend a major problem. It is difficult to get started in the morning and the time between procedures is also quite long. On top of this our department is part of the center for robotic surgery in the capital region of Copenhagen, and this in itself actually also decrease effectiveness in the operating department. The reason is, that it does take some time to set-up the robots in the morning and change time also seems to be a little longer than if things were running smoothly.

It is certainly not easy to solve such a problem and I guess the only way forward will be to have very firm support from the hospital management and a signal to the entire staff that if we do not produce more than we used to then people will simply have to look for another job. I know that this may not be in line with modern management theories where it is better to coach the staff to change the behavior by themselves, but I can assure you that we have tried almost everything through the years. The situation is not fully solved yet, but it is already running better than a year ago.

13 ROOM CHANGES

In order to signal a clearly defined top management in the department and a visible management team, we moved offices so that all the administrative people including the head surgeon and head nurse would have offices located very closely together. This is together with the head of the secretaries, the operation planner, people looking after the economy etc.

14 ECONOMY – PROBLEMS AND SOLUTIONS

For 2012 the department had to reduce costs for about 2 mill US$ but when I started February 1st, 2012 many of these cuts had not been implemented.

It soon became obvious that many of the planned reductions could actually not go through, because especially the surgical staff on call simply had too much work to do all evening and all night to be able to reduce the on call personnel as planned. Furthermore, the situation in general for the payment for extra hours for the surgeons was almost a catastrophe where we paid around 90.000 US$ every month in total to the surgeons for extra hours. Furthermore, after a few months one of the surgeons told us that the department actually owned him about 85.000 US$ for extra hours going 4 years back in time. We did not know anything about this and this extra deficit therefore had to be absorbed in the 2012 budget. We had to implement a new system for electronic patient files where we did not get any compensation from the directors. This constituted about 30.000 US$

for extra computer equipment and about a half year working time for teaching of staff.

The medical section received a quite good payment for on call although they almost never came in to the hospital in the evening or night hours. With only 14 beds and very few acute admissions in the medical section we chose to change their on call schedule and thereby save some money.

Finally, in the merging of the endoscopy units where we received a full endoscopy unit from another hospital, the negotiations had not been performed well up to the merger by the previous administration because we simply did not get the budget that we should. So also in this area we had a deficit to begin with.

The main problem seemed to be the lack of control of the spending for extra hours for surgeons. We therefore very quickly decided to hire a controller to look at this on a daily basis. This person is very skilled in the work planning system and we have given him full authority to decide who can come in on extra days and who cannot. It is very important to give this guy full power and responsibility and it has resulted in a remarkable reduction in our spending for extra hours for surgeons.

It was not easy for the surgeons to accept that a non-medical person could actually decide if they should come in or not, but the head nurse and me have signaled without any doubt that it had to be this way. He also controls the number of days that consultants in both the surgical and medical section can be away for congresses and other external activities and only if there is doubt the top management gets involved.

To hire this guy for controlling our spending was of course initially an additional spending, but it has turned out to be an extremely good investment for our department.

15 WHAT CAN THEY EXPECT FROM ME?

Since I am both university professor and head of a department with normal clinical consultant responsibilities it is not possible for me to be very active in the normal clinical work in the department. By rules I have to spend at least 50% of my time for university tasks (research and teaching) and when I also have to of course spend quite a lot of time at meetings with directors and other department heads etc., there is certainly not much time left for normal clinical work. The result is therefore that I am present almost every morning for the morning meeting and I perform special surgical procedures 1-2 days/month. This is of course not very much, but there is simply not time enough for more at the moment.

Perhaps when the department has gone through all the restructuring, then the administrative side may be less, and there will be more time for clinical work. I am also responsible for a large research unit in the department consisting of approximately 20 full time researchers and we publish around

40 scientific papers per year where I am deeply involved in the process from idea through protocol, data analysis and critical revision of the papers.

The only solution for making this work was to appoint a dedicated chief of surgery and a dedicated chief of gastroenterology in the department. These two guys have full power to change staffing on a daily basis and to plan the daily activities so that things get done. Below these two chiefs of surgery and gastroenterology there are dedicated team leaders in every team consisting of a surgeon or physician and a department nurse. These teams have their own budgets so that they have to look at both spending and income for their specific section.

16 TIME PLAN FOR THE NEW DEPARTMENT

Very early it was communicated to the entire department that they could not expect to see me doing lots of clinical work for a while. We had enormous economically problems and they should expect that this would take up to perhaps a year to develop a plan and have things running smoothly.

After this economical recovery the next phase would be to look at new developments in patient care, education and research. This is of course not all true because it is not possible to implement drastic economical changes without looking at innovation at the same time, but it was formulated this way just to signal that there would be a long period in the beginning where the head nurse and I would dedicate time almost fully to economical recovery, and after this we would go into other areas of the administrative tasks.

During this process we have said again and again that the goal was to make our department the best in our country both for patients and for staff and we will never give up on this ultimate goal.

17 PRODUCTION AND INNOVATION

The activity in an academic department is naturally divided into three blocks consisting of diagnosis and treatment (or you can call it patient care), education, and research. All three areas are important and we cannot cut down on one and still look ourselves in the mirror and say that we are running a high-end academic department.

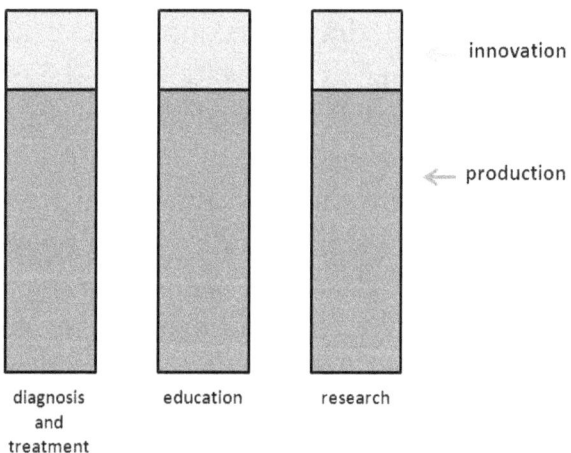

In every area there is activity that you could

call basic production – things that we are simply just doing on a daily basis and with a good quality. However, in our monthly meetings with the team leaders in the different teams we are explicitly asking them to think further on and to develop innovation strategies in patient care, education and research.

This means that in all the areas of the department there has to be new developments in all three areas. This has several aims. First of all of course it will drive new development in the department which in itself is natural and a must in a big academic unit. However, there is also another indirect effect, and that is that when we signal to the team leaders that they are actually allowed to invent new things, then suddenly fantastic new ideas will come up and it will indeed motivate and inspire the staff to be happy at work. It will give everybody a feeling of having influence. And why shouldn't new development come from the staff on the floor? – They know what is happening and of course they are the ones who should develop these new ideas. The management will provide necessary support for different new innovations.

You may think that it is a bit risky because it may cost more money, but in fact it most often would reduce costs because the staff is surprisingly very much aware that the things cannot cost more. Thus, they quite naturally think in lean principles and suggest smarter ways of doing things.

18 IT IS OK TO BE THE BEST

Once a famous statesman said: "I am easily satisfied with the very best". We have worked on creating a mind-set in all the staffs that it is actually OK to be the best in certain clinical areas. It is not possible to be the best in every area of a scientific department, but why not focus and talk about the areas where we are actually some of the best in the country.

We have not had time yet to give this our full focus but in the near future we will start to organize international symposia in the different clinical areas where we are very good, and we will cultivate both the production and innovation part of patient care and patient research especially in these clinical areas.

Nowadays it is important to have a branding strategy for an academically active department and it of course should be focused on clinical areas where we are very good. Currently, the clinical areas in focus are endoscopy, laparoscopic surgery, robotic surgery, ultrasound, inflammatory bowel disease, hepatitis, anal cancer, recurrent rectal cancer and hernias.

19 NEW PROFESSORS AND OTHER ACADEMIC PERSONS

Currently, the department has one full (no time limit) professor in minimal invasive surgery, one 5-year professor in endoscopy, one 5-year professor in inflammatory bowel disease and a visiting professor in endo-microscopy which is an advanced endoscopic procedure. We hope very soon also to employ a 5-year professor in e-health with focus on inflammatory bowel disease and other gastroenterological diseases and a 5-year professor in perioperative optimization.

In this way most of our clinical areas are covered by academic staff which is necessary to drive especially the research part of the activity.

20 FINANCIAL RECOVERY - WHAT HAVE WE DONE?

As described previously there were major problems both with expenses and income. It was therefore obvious that no single intervention would solve the problems and we therefore had to develop a recovery plan covering both expenses and income.

Expenses

The previous management has had the wrong impression that if some of the intern or residents positions were not filled, then the department would save money. This is actually the exact contrary because if somebody is missing in the on-call layer, then the others have to cover, and this will create overtime that has to be paid as 50% plus to the normal salary. All together it is therefore more expensive not to have the positions filled than to have them filled with residents and interns. One of the first things we did was therefore to fill the available positions in the department.

Previously the consultants came in in their spare time/days off if they wanted to participate in special operations. They did not ask permissions to do this, but they just came in and got payment for these extra days. Now we normally plan the procedures on the days where the dedicated surgeons are actually working and thereby it is not anymore allowed or necessary to come in on days off.

From the very beginning we have articulated the economical problems at every given opportunity. This has created awareness that we have a common problem that has to be solved. If we do not solve the problem with the economy, then everything else cannot function since we have to cut down to an extend that new development will not be possible.

As mentioned previously we employed a controller to look after expenses and work planning for the surgical and medical doctors. This has been very effective and the investment in spending his extra salary has been more than worth while.

Every month we look at the numbers for expenses both for salary and for other costs. If there is a sudden increase then we dissect the numbers in order to find out what has happened.

We have appointed team leaders in all the different teams in the department and they have delegated the responsibility so that spending follows the monthly budget. This has been very successful especially in the nursing group, where monthly spending has been under very good control.

Income

Hospital health care in our country is run by diagnosis related groups (DRG) and everything we do has a certain value and we have to produce a certain amount of income every month. As for the expenses we also follow the DRG income on a monthly basis and if numbers are decreasing then we make a prompt plan to change this.

Example: At one point we saw that the day clinic in the medical section had decreased income and after a detailed analysis it turned out that many patients did not come as planned. Because of this the team leaders for the medical day clinic developed a plan where reminders were sent out ahead of every visit and patients got a reminder also as a text message on their cell phones if they had given their permission for this.

Another example: It was very early obvious that we did not produce enough income for surgical operations and a detailed analysis showed that the problem were lying in not doing enough hernia operations and operations for gallstone disease. It was obvious that the problem was actually not having enough operative capacity, but that we had too long waiting time for the first visit in the surgical day clinic. In order to overcome this we decided to have extra days with opening in the evening hours (this is not normal) and the investment in extra salary both for nurses and surgeons was easily counteracted by the increased income for extra operations. Forward we have increased the capacity in the surgical day clinic especially for hernias and gallbladders in order to have a higher income for the department.

21 WHAT IS NEXT?

To begin with it was communicated very clearly that there were several phases in the new department administration and development. The first phase was naturally to get control of the economy of the department since there were major problems both on the expenses and income side. It was clearly stated that this could not be solved over night and that the staff should expect a period of up to a year before this was under control.

After this then all the different teams in the department would start working seriously with production and innovation for patient care, education and research. Thus, the next phase of the department is actually now ongoing and we have initiated team meetings with all the different teams where we discuss and plan activity within patient care, education and research, and with a firm focus on innovation along with the normal production.

All the teams are offered a full day of discussion/planning at a remote location in order to develop the necessary plans for the coming years.

22 SUMMARY OF CHANGES IN THE NEW DEPARTMENT

In summary, the first year has been filled with a lot of activity and we have focused specifically on the following:

- Clear mission statement
- Develop a clear management hierarchy
- Delegating responsibility and local management to team leaders
- Create possibility for discussing difficult cases every day
- Various interventions to increase patient satisfaction
- Restructuring of the day clinics to have more patients
- Merging of three endoscopy units into one
- New organization of acute functions
- Better planning of operations in order to increase production
- Change of offices in order to make a defined management area in the department
- To hire a controller in order to get

better control of spending especially for the surgeons' salaries
- Appointing a chief of surgery and a chief of gastroenterology for the daily management in the two sections
- Defining and articulating the three important areas 1) patient care, 2) education, and 3) research, and that everybody has to think innovation on top of production
- Define and nourish our areas of great expertise and develop a branding strategy for these
- Cover all these areas of expertise with academic professors in order to support research and development in these areas
- Fill available positions as residents and interns
- Change of operative planning so that the correct operations are booked on days where the correct surgeons are working
- Follow expenses as well as income on a monthly basis and as soon as thing tend to go wrong then develop prompt interventions
- Create a general awareness in all parts

of the department that we have had major economic problems and that as soon as this has been solved we will focus on all the other areas in order to make our department one of the best in the country

23 CONCLUSION

The past year has been very busy and also very interesting. It has been a kind of a rebirth of a large academic department at a university hospital and we have during the first year especially struggled with a lot of economical problems. I am very proud to be able to say, that we actually came out of 2012 for the first time in more than 10 years with black numbers on the bottom line instead of red numbers. This has only been possible because many things have been changed simultaneously and the staff has all been aware of the strategy and in agreement with the plans. Everybody has worked very hard to achieve this fantastic goal and we are now able to look ahead and to develop plans for changes in patient care, research and education.

I would have loved a year ago to be able to read a book like this in order to get some tips and tricks, and I hope that the book can be helpful for new leaders of big departments where there are similar problems.

Most of the interventions that we have done are not at all rocket science but merely common sense. I do actually feel it to be a little refreshing that it does not require long education in management to be able to implement a rebirth and restructuring of a big unit like ours and actually to achieve balance in what looked like a catastrophic economical situation just a year ago. Many of the interventions described in this book can probably also be applied to other hospital departments or other sections in health care.

24 THANK YOU

I want to thank you for staying on to the very end of this book, and if you have time I would very much appreciate if you could post a short review and your opinion about what you have read.

25 FURTHER READING

1. Souba WW, Wilmore DW. Judging surgical research: How should we evaluate performance and measure value? Ann Surg 232:1;32-41.

2. Schwartz RW, Pogge C. Physician leadership is essential to the survival of teaching hospitals. Am J Surg 2000;179:462-468.

3. Schwartz RW, Pogge C. Physician leadership: essential skills in a changing environment. Am J Surg 2000;180:187-192.

4. Warren OJ, Carnall R. Medical leadership: why it's important, what is required, and how we develop it. Postgrad Med J 2011;87:27-32.

5. Tomlinson C, LaBossière, Rommens K, Birch DW. The Canadian general surgery resident: defining current challenges for surgical leadership. J Can Chir 2012;55:S184-S190.

6. Goldman EF, Wesner M, Karnchanomai O. Implementing the leadership development. Plans of faculty education fellows: a structured approach. Acad Med 2012;87:1177-1184.

7. Mallon WT, Buckley PF. The current state and future possibilities of recruiting leaders of academic health centers. Acad Med 2012; 87: 1171-1176.

8. Haizlip J, May N, Schorling J, Williams A, Plews-Ogan M. The negative bias, medical education, and the culture of academic medicine: why culture change is hard. Acad Med 2012;87:1205-1209.

9. Souba WW. The 3 essential responsibilities. Arch Surg 2010;145:540-543.

10. Turnipseed WD, Lund DP, Sollenberger D. Product line development. A strategy for clinical success in Academic centers. Ann Surg 2007;246:585-592.

ABOUT THE AUTHOR

Jacob Rosenberg (1964) was born and grew up in Copenhagen, Denmark. He is professor of surgery at the University of Copenhagen, and department head at the department of surgery, Herlev Hospital (also in Copenhagen). He has published more than 400 scientific papers in research journals, and several book chapters in surgery and related areas. He is currently editor of the Journal of the Danish Medical Association and the Danish Medical Journal, and sits in the International Committee of Medical Journal Editors.

www.ingramcontent.com/pod-product-compliance
Lightning Source LLC
Chambersburg PA
CBHW071636170526
45166CB00003B/1335